KEEP ON TRACK BY KEEPING TRACK!

E x e r c i s e   L o g

Activinotes

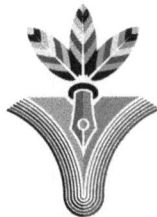

Activinotes

DAILY JOURNALS, PLANNERS, NOTEBOOKS AND OTHER BLANK BOOKS

Date:_____

Aerobic /Cardio

Exercises	Time/ Distance	Intensity	Calories Burned

Strenght

Exercises	Sets/ Rep	Weight	Rest

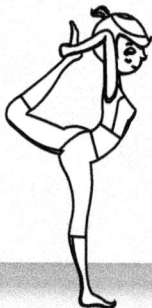

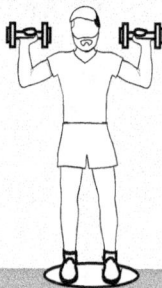

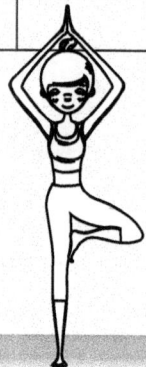

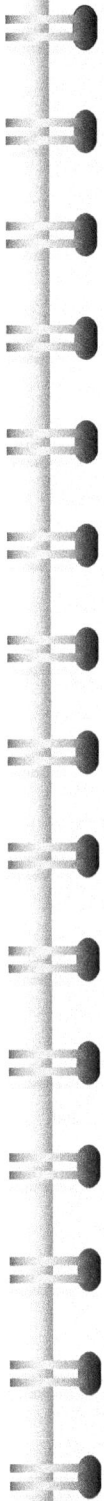

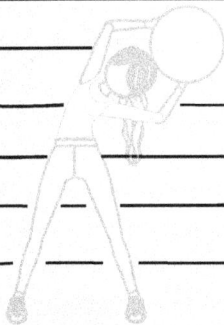

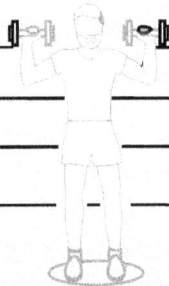

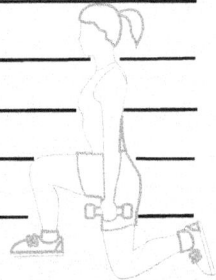

Date:_____

Aerobic /Cardio

Exercises	Time/ Distance	Intensity	Calories Burned

Strenght

Exercises	Sets/ Rep	Weight	Rest

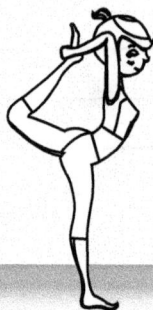

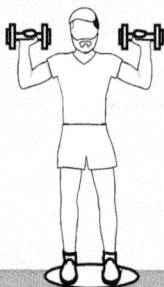

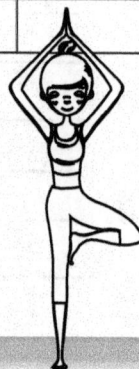

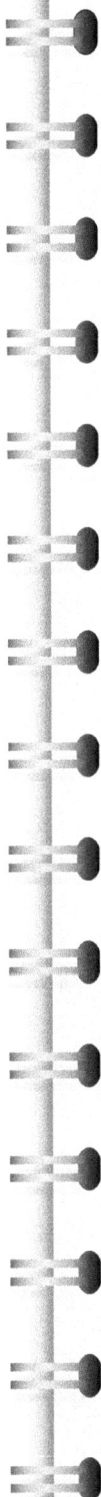

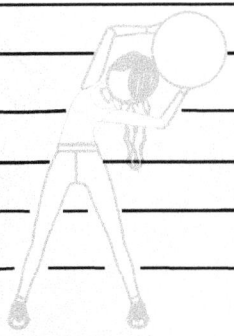

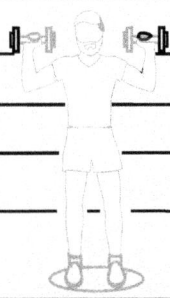

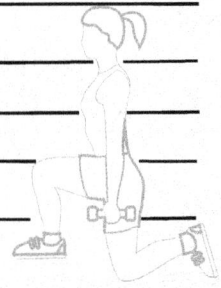

Date:_____

Aerobic / Cardio

Exercises	Time/ Distance	Intensity	Calories Burned

Strenght

Exercises	Sets/ Rep	Weight	Rest

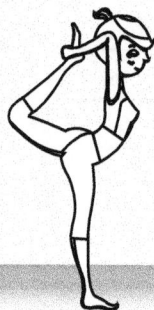

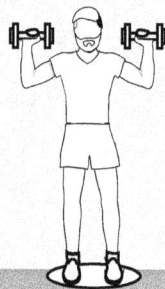

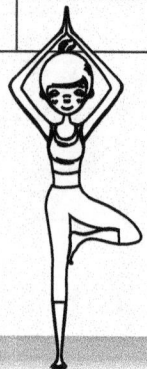

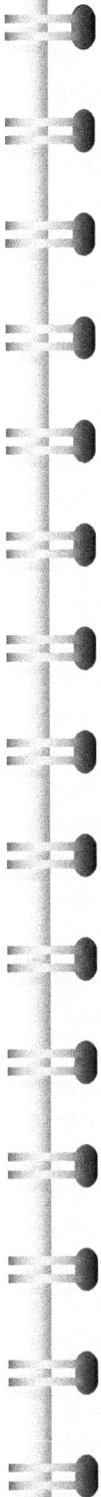

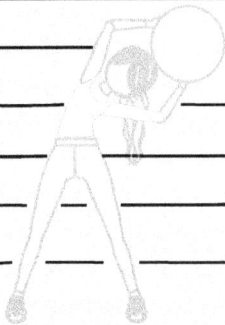

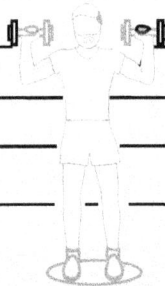

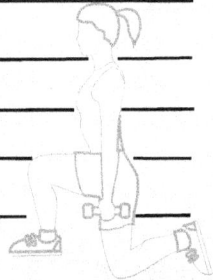

Date:_____

Aerobic / Cardio

Exercises	Time/ Distance	Intensity	Calories Burned

Strenght

Exercises	Sets/ Rep	Weight	Rest

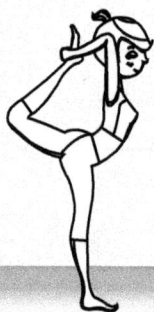

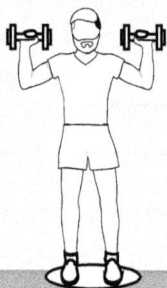

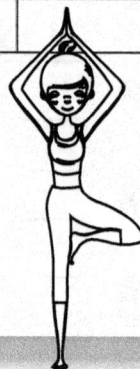

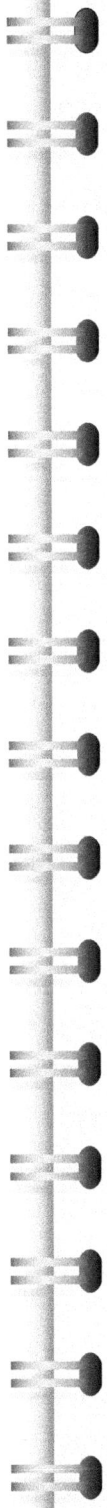

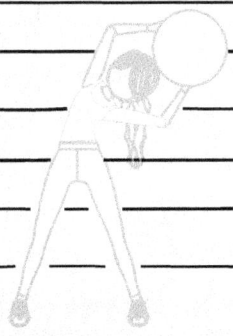

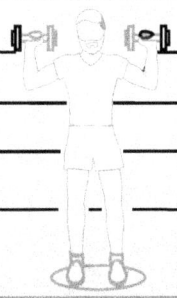

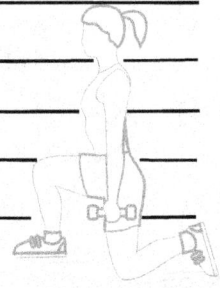

Date:_____

Aerobic /Cardio

Exercises	Time/ Distance	Intensity	Calories Burned

Strenght

Exercises	Sets/ Rep	Weight	Rest

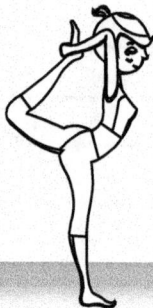

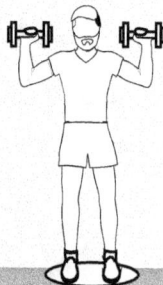

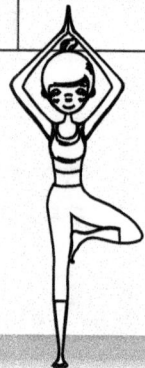

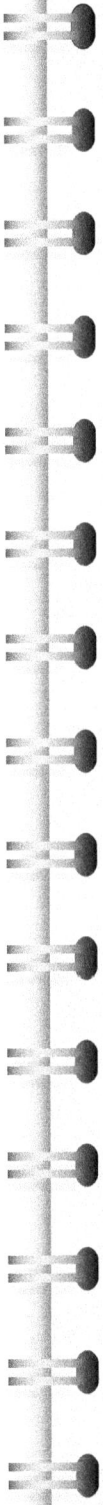

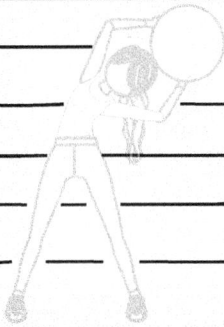

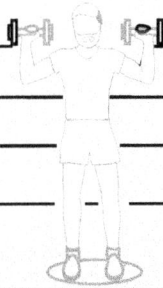

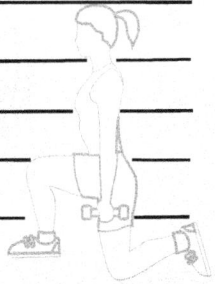

Date:_____

Aerobic /Cardio

Exercises	Time/ Distance	Intensity	Calories Burned

Strenght

Exercises	Sets/ Rep	Weight	Rest

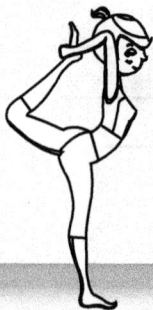

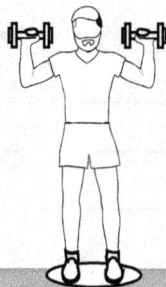

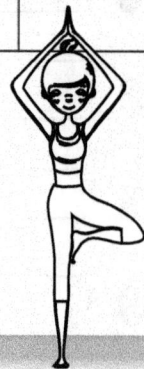

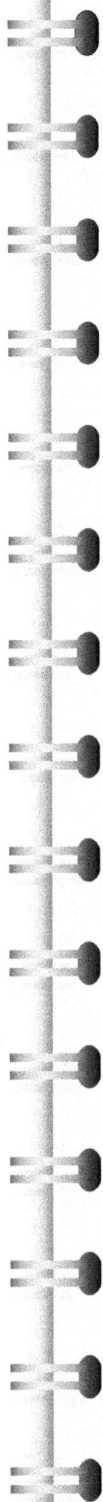

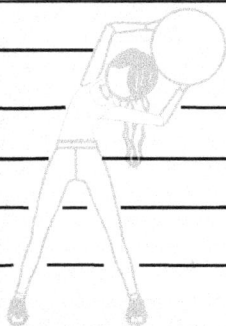

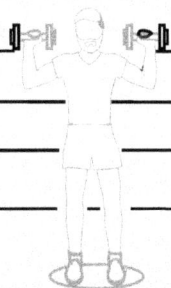

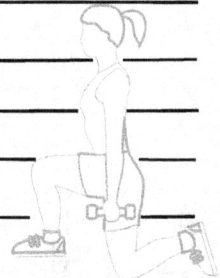

Date:_____

Aerobic / Cardio

Exercises	Time/ Distance	Intensity	Calories Burned

Strenght

Exercises	Sets/ Rep	Weight	Rest

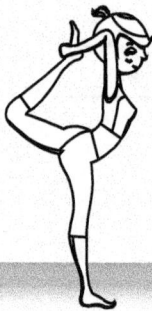

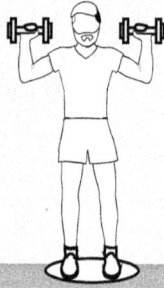

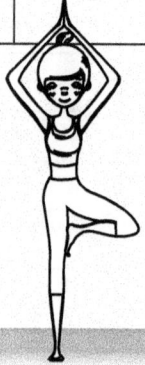

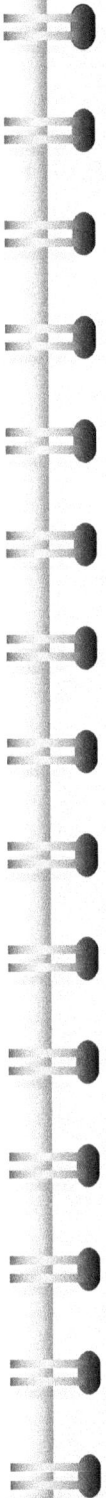

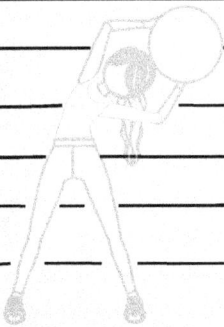

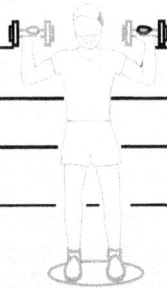

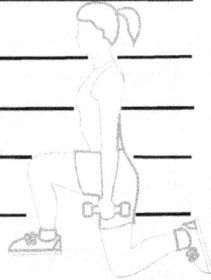

Date:_____

Aerobic /Cardio

Exercises	Time/ Distance	Intensity	Calories Burned

Strenght

Exercises	Sets/ Rep	Weight	Rest

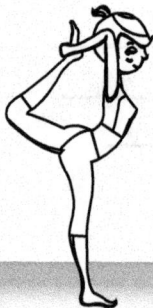

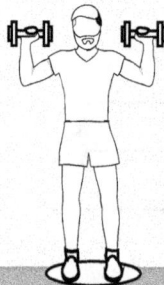

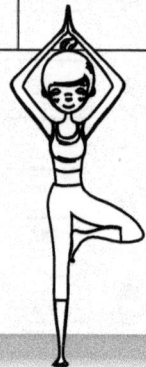

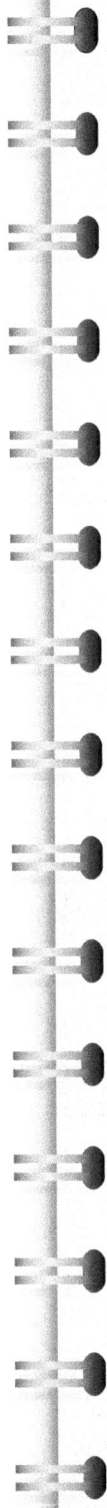

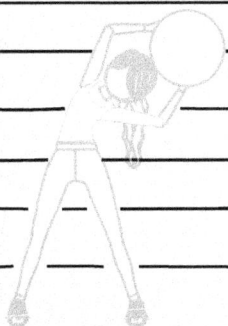

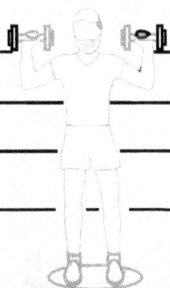

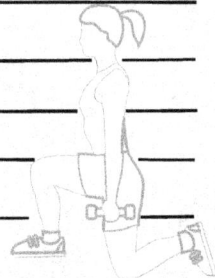

Date:_____

Aerobic / Cardio

Exercises	Time/ Distance	Intensity	Calories Burned

Strenght

Exercises	Sets/ Rep	Weight	Rest

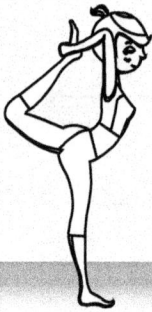

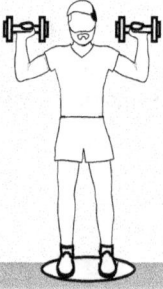

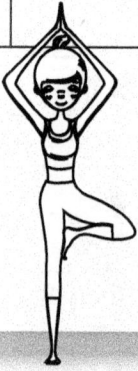

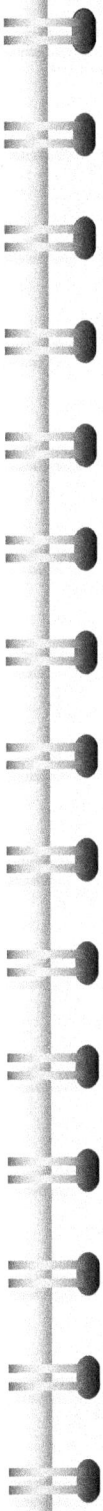

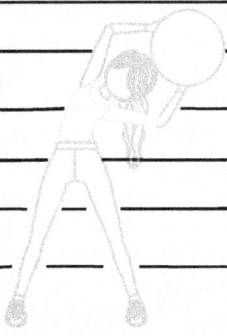

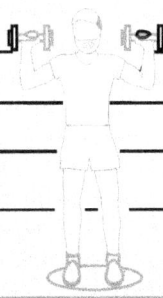

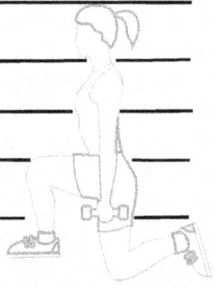

Date:_____

Aerobic /Cardio

Exercises	Time/ Distance	Intensity	Calories Burned

Strenght

Exercises	Sets/ Rep	Weight	Rest

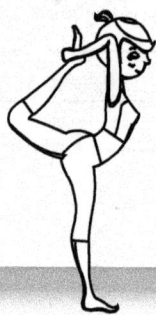

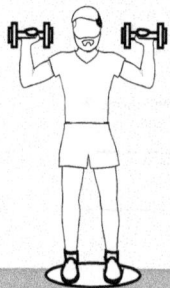

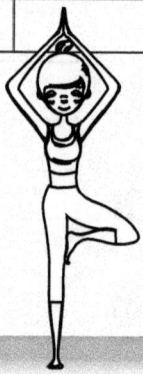

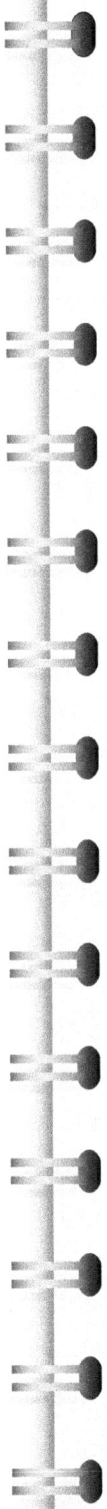

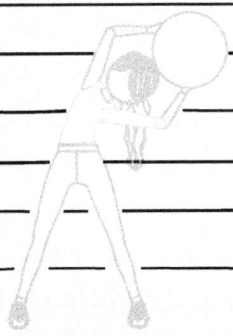

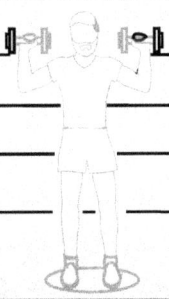

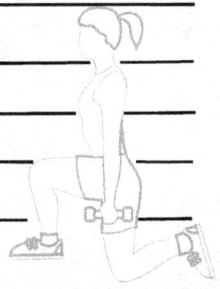

Date:_____

Aerobic /Cardio

Exercises	Time/ Distance	Intensity	Calories Burned

Strenght

Exercises	Sets/ Rep	Weight	Rest

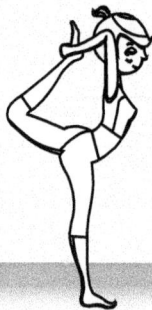

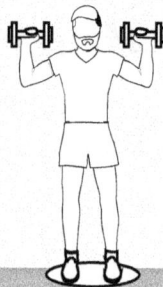

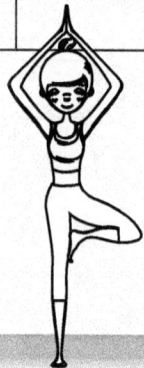

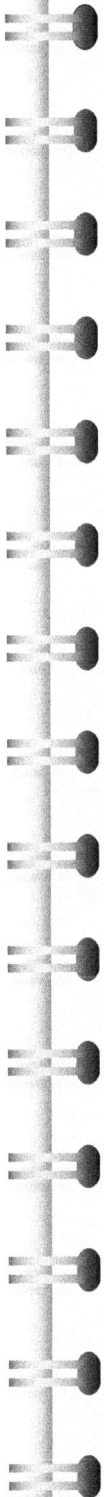

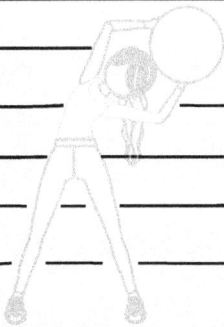

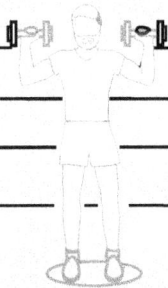

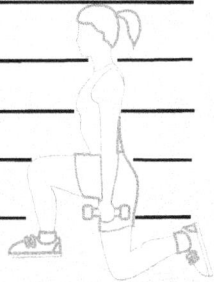

Date:_____

Aerobic /Cardio

Exercises	Time/ Distance	Intensity	Calories Burned

Strenght

Exercises	Sets/ Rep	Weight	Rest

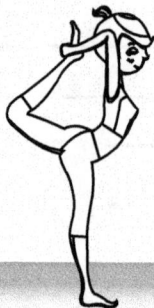

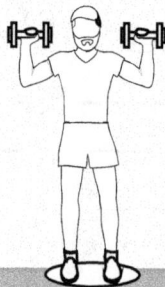

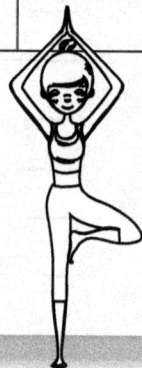

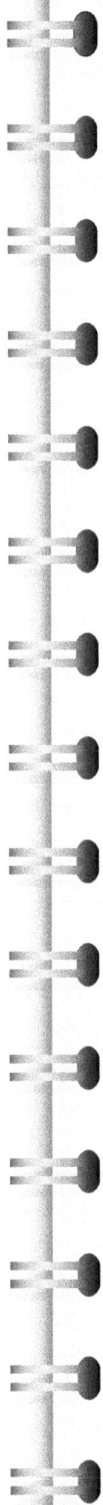

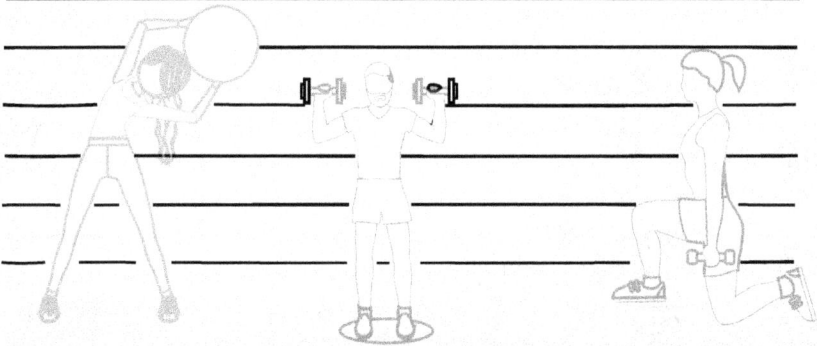

Date:_____

Aerobic /Cardio

Exercises	Time/ Distance	Intensity	Calories Burned

Strenght

Exercises	Sets/ Rep	Weight	Rest

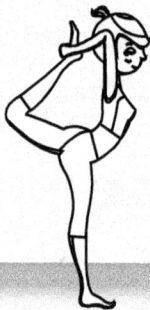

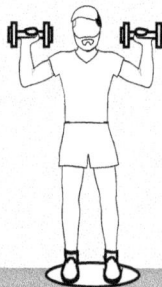

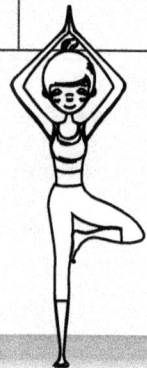

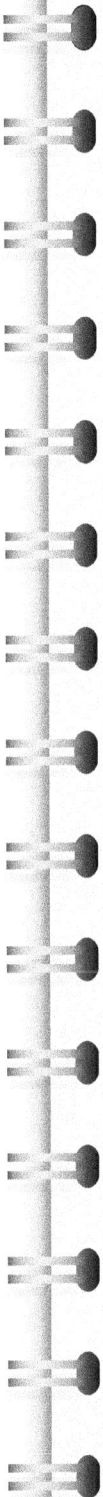

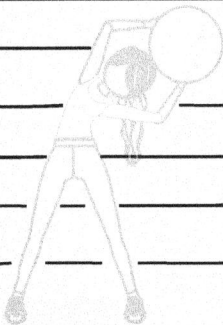

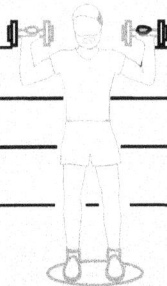

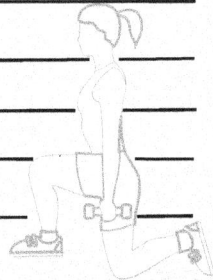

Date:_____

Aerobic /Cardio

Exercises	Time/ Distance	Intensity	Calories Burned

Strenght

Exercises	Sets/ Rep	Weight	Rest

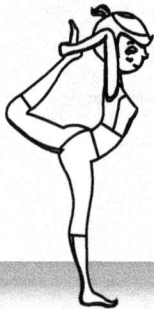

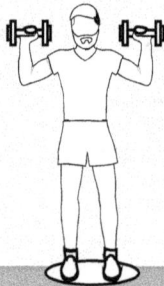

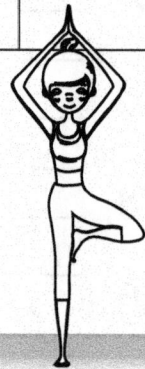

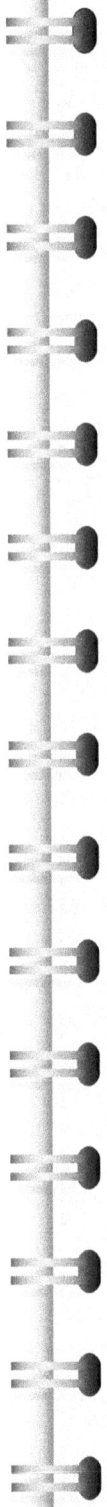

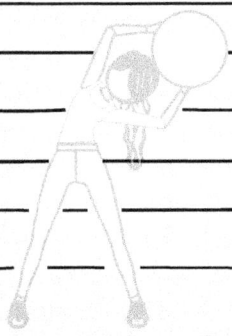

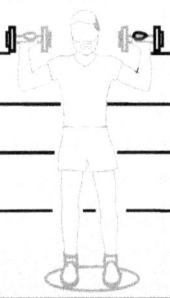

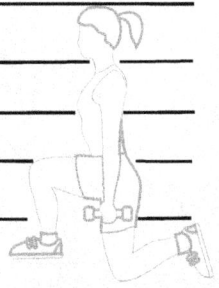

Date:_____

Aerobic /Cardio

Exercises	Time/ Distance	Intensity	Calories Burned

Strenght

Exercises	Sets/ Rep	Weight	Rest

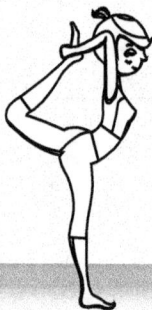

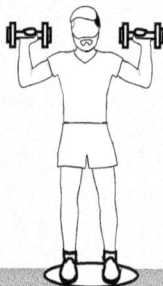

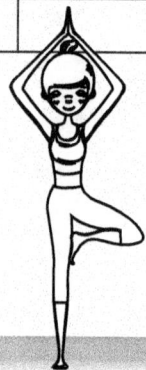

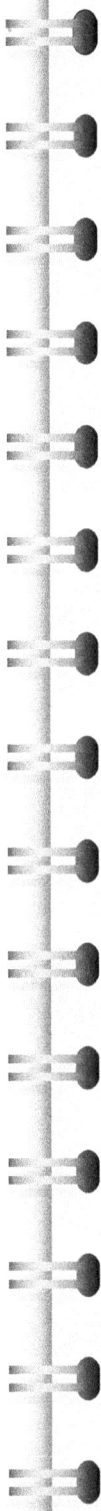

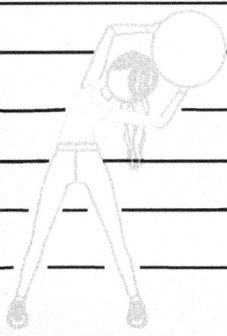

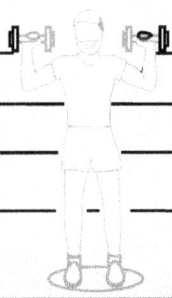

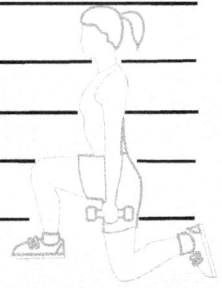

Date:_____

Aerobic /Cardio

Exercises	Time/ Distance	Intensity	Calories Burned

Strenght

Exercises	Sets/ Rep	Weight	Rest

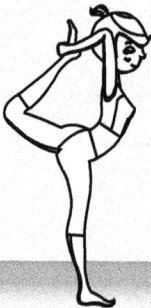

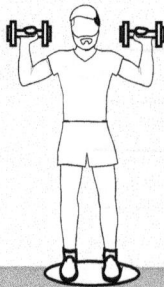

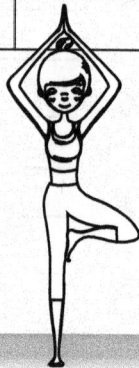

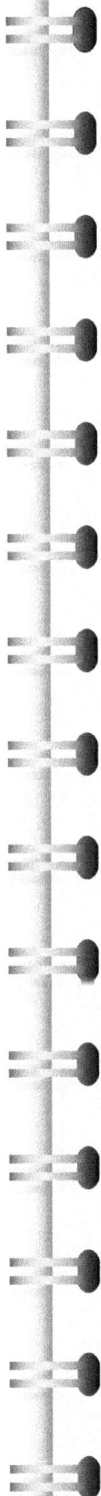

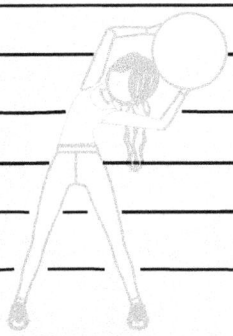

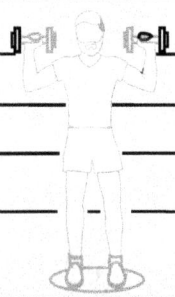

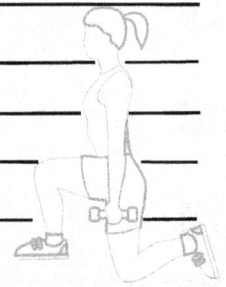

Date:_____

Aerobic /Cardio			
Exercises	Time/ Distance	Intensity	Calories Burned

Strenght			
Exercises	Sets/ Rep	Weight	Rest

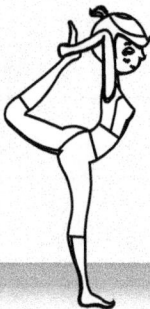

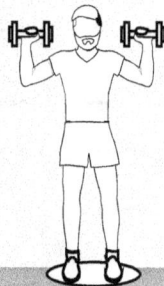

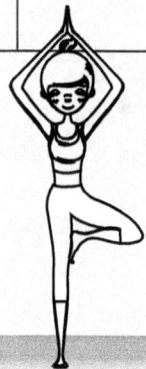

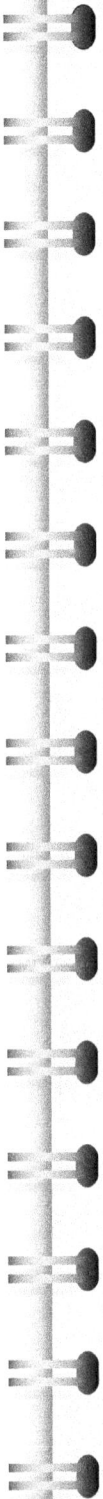

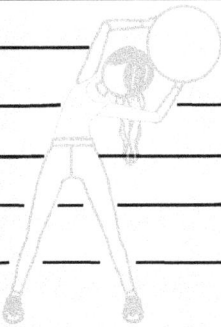

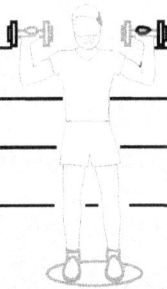

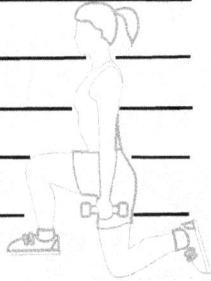

Date:_____

Aerobic / Cardio

Exercises	Time/ Distance	Intensity	Calories Burned

Strenght

Exercises	Sets/ Rep	Weight	Rest

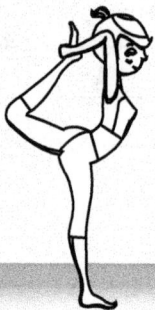

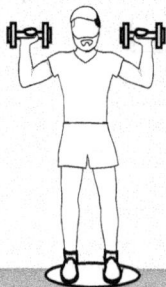

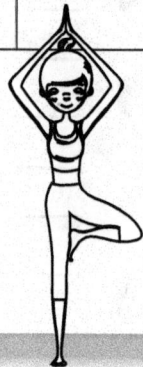

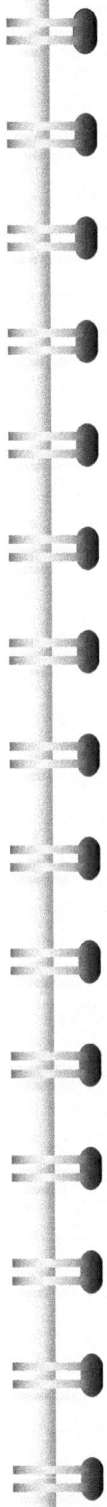

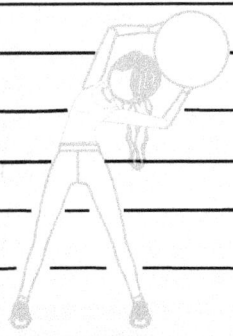

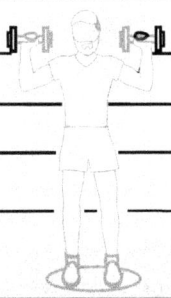

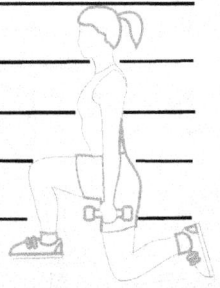

Date:_____

Aerobic /Cardio

Exercises	Time/ Distance	Intensity	Calories Burned

Strenght

Exercises	Sets/ Rep	Weight	Rest

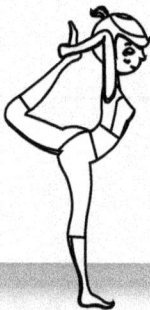

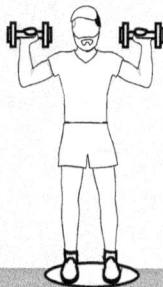

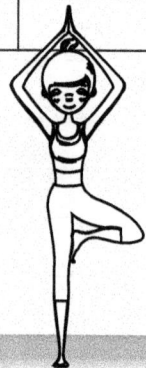

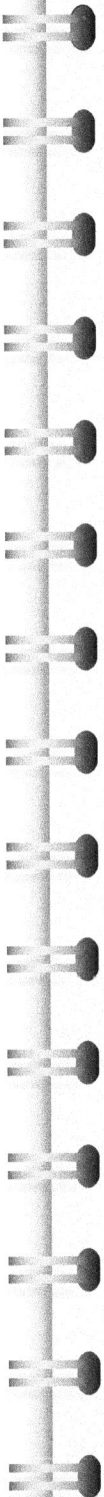

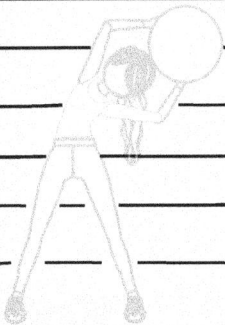

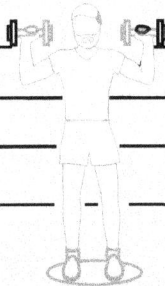

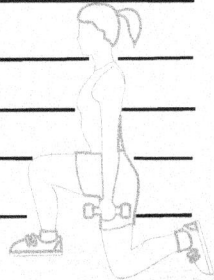

Date:_____

Aerobic /Cardio

Exercises	Time/ Distance	Intensity	Calories Burned

Strenght

Exercises	Sets/ Rep	Weight	Rest

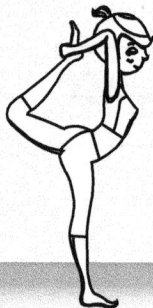

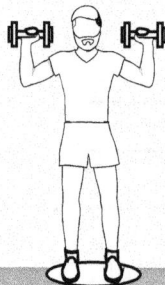

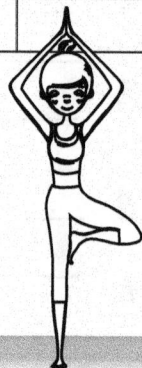

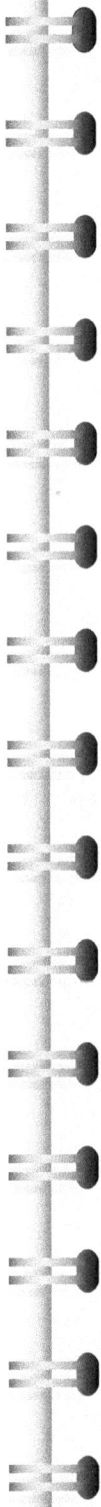

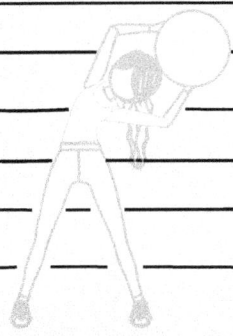

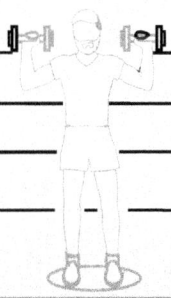

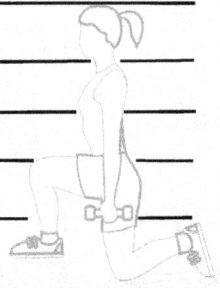

Date:_____

Aerobic /Cardio

Exercises	Time/ Distance	Intensity	Calories Burned

Strenght

Exercises	Sets/ Rep	Weight	Rest

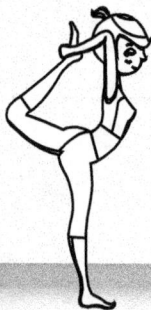

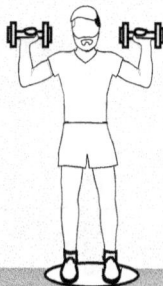

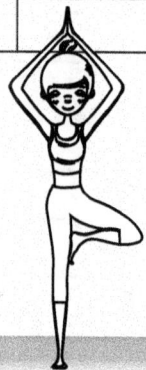

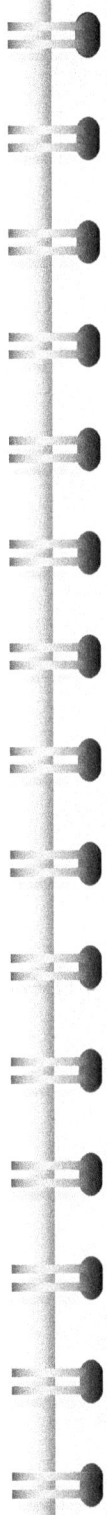

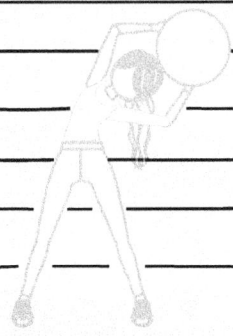

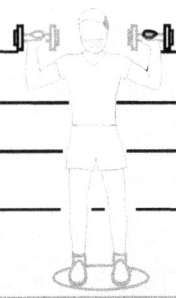

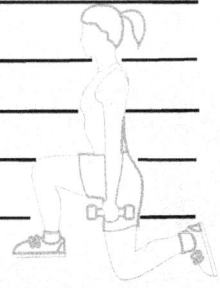

Date:_____

Aerobic /Cardio

Exercises	Time/ Distance	Intensity	Calories Burned

Strenght

Exercises	Sets/ Rep	Weight	Rest

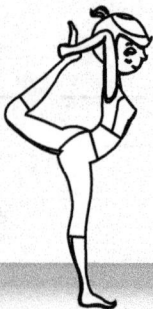

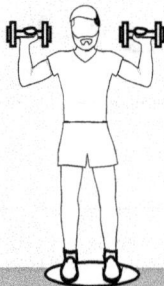

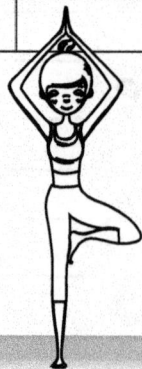

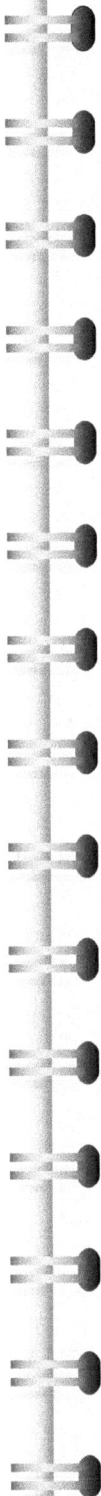

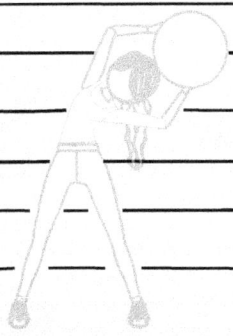

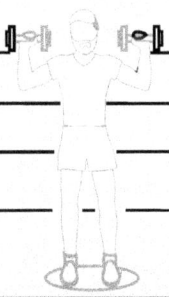

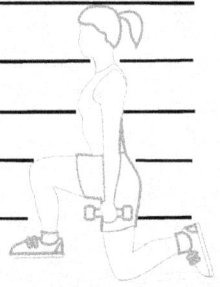

Date:_____

Aerobic /Cardio

Exercises	Time/ Distance	Intensity	Calories Burned

Strenght

Exercises	Sets/ Rep	Weight	Rest

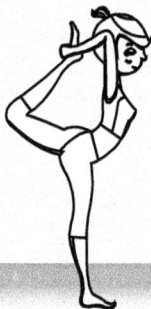

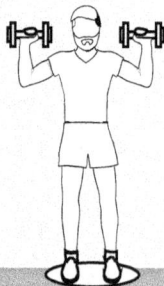

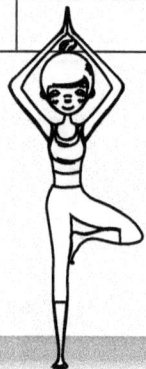

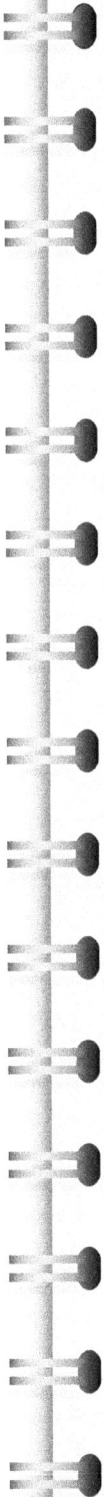

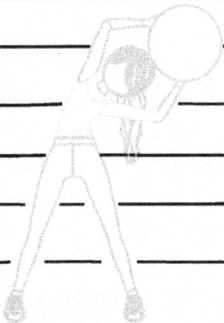

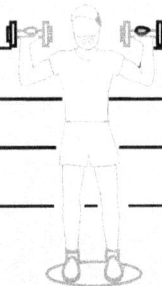

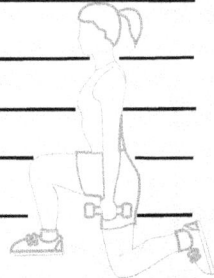

Date:_____

Aerobic /Cardio

Exercises	Time/ Distance	Intensity	Calories Burned

Strenght

Exercises	Sets/ Rep	Weight	Rest

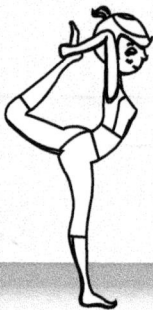

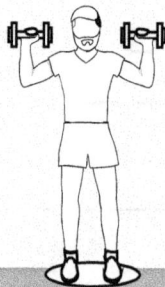

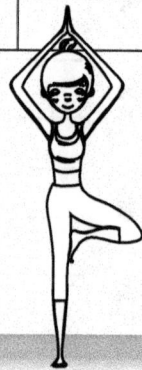

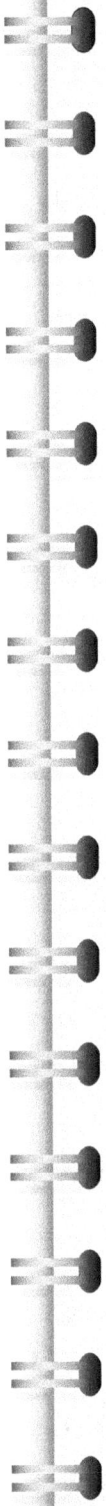

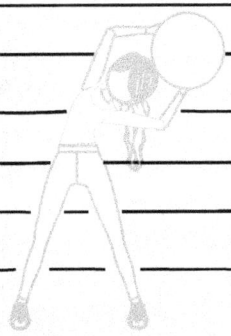

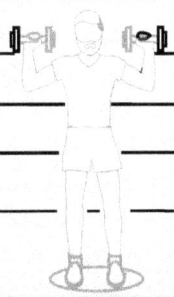

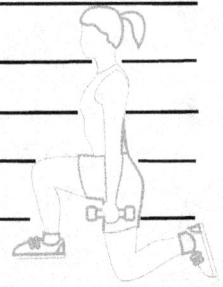

Date:_____

Aerobic / Cardio

Exercises	Time/ Distance	Intensity	Calories Burned

Strenght

Exercises	Sets/ Rep	Weight	Rest

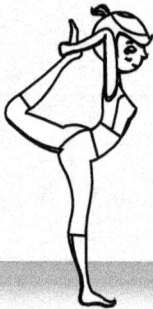

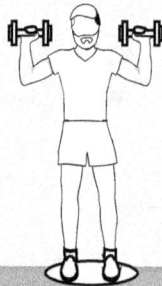

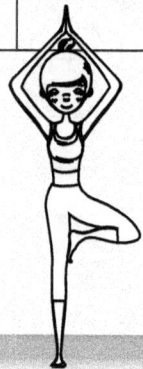

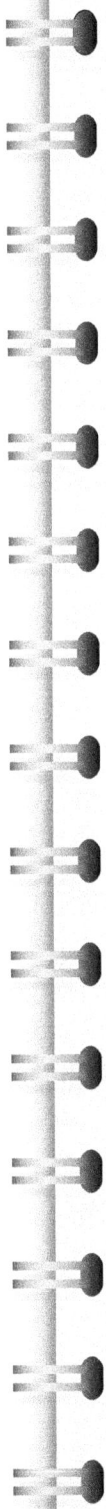

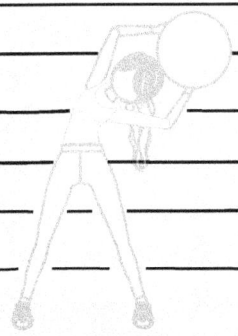

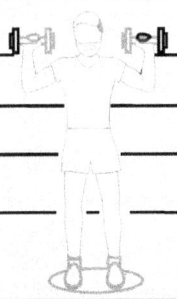

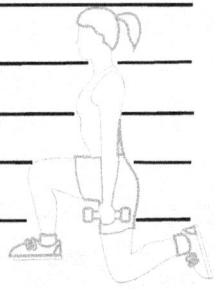

Date:_____

Aerobic /Cardio

Exercises	Time/ Distance	Intensity	Calories Burned

Strenght

Exercises	Sets/ Rep	Weight	Rest

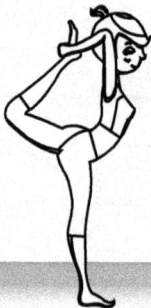

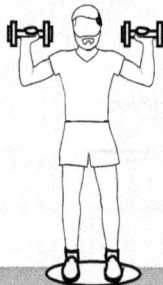

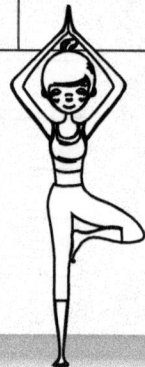

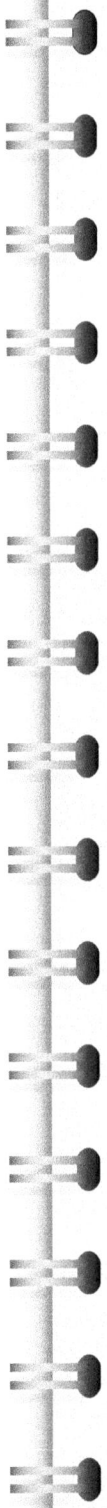

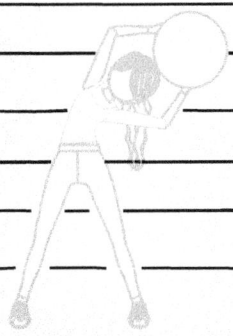

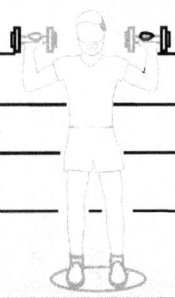

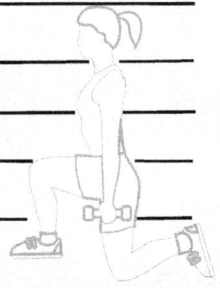

Date:_____

Aerobic /Cardio

Exercises	Time/ Distance	Intensity	Calories Burned

Strenght

Exercises	Sets/ Rep	Weight	Rest

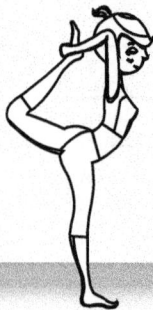

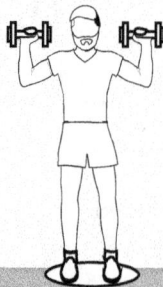

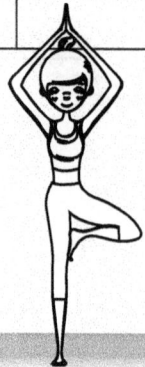

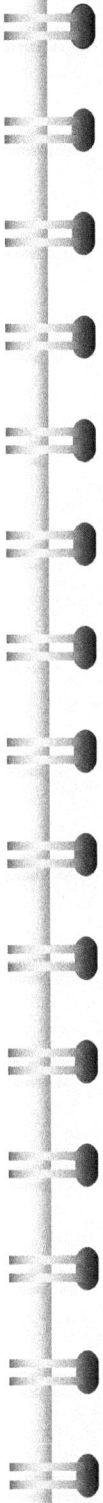

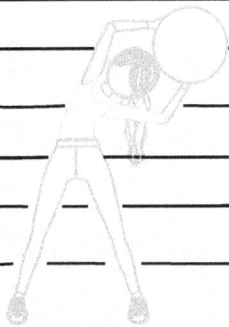

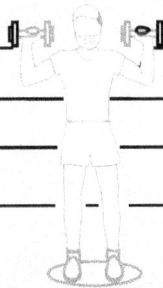

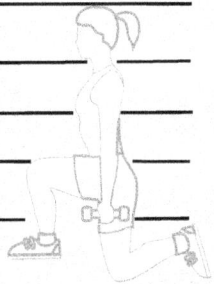

Date:_____

Aerobic / Cardio

Exercises	Time/ Distance	Intensity	Calories Burned

Strenght

Exercises	Sets/ Rep	Weight	Rest

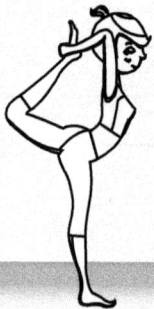

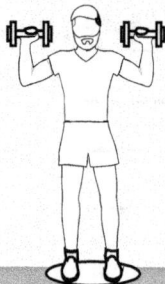

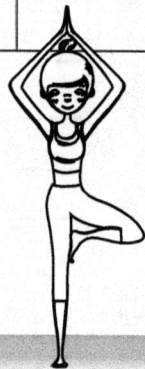

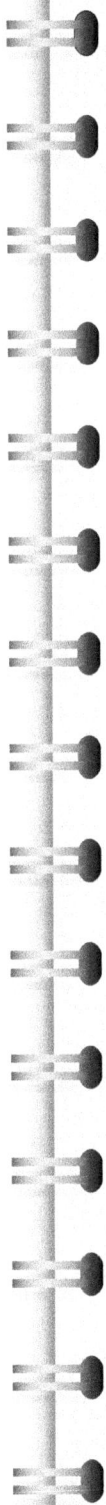

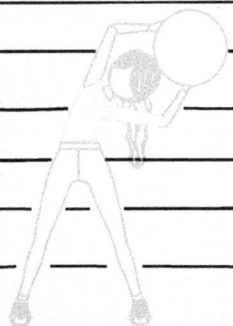

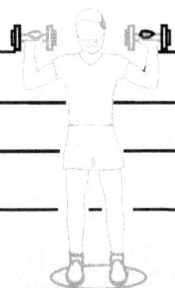

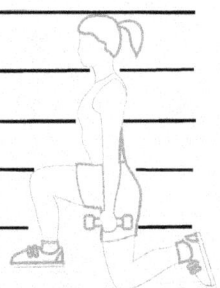

Date:_____

Aerobic /Cardio

Exercises	Time/ Distance	Intensity	Calories Burned

Strenght

Exercises	Sets/ Rep	Weight	Rest

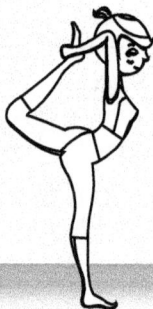

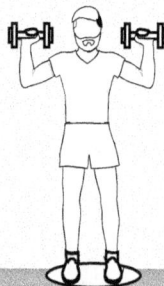

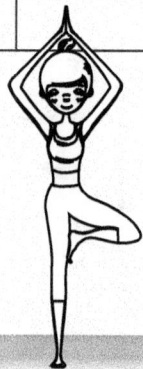

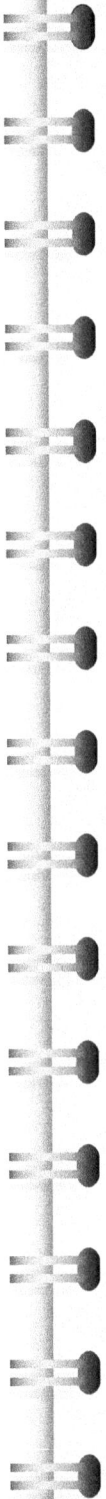

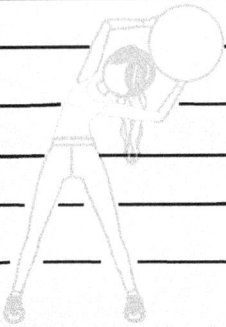

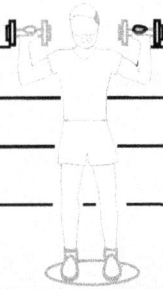

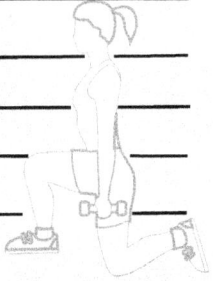

Date:_____

Aerobic /Cardio

Exercises	Time/ Distance	Intensity	Calories Burned

Strenght

Exercises	Sets/ Rep	Weight	Rest

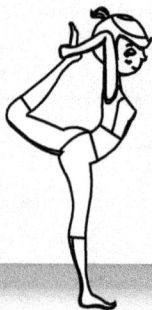

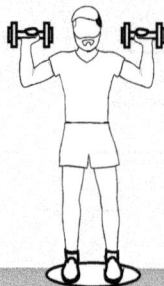

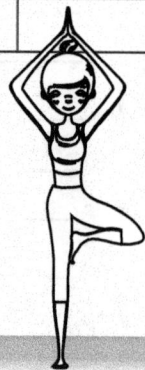

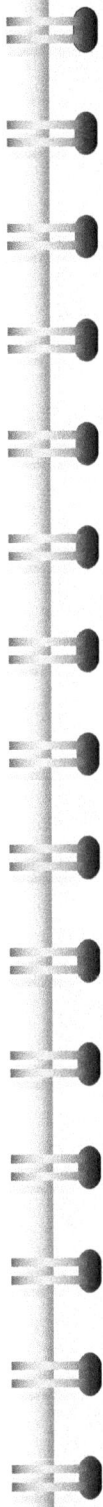

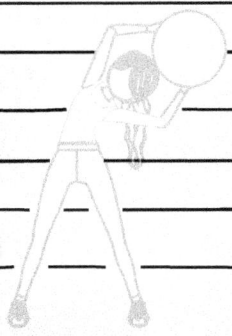

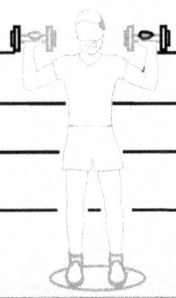

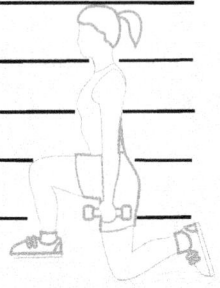

Date:_____

Aerobic / Cardio

Exercises	Time/ Distance	Intensity	Calories Burned

Strenght

Exercises	Sets/ Rep	Weight	Rest

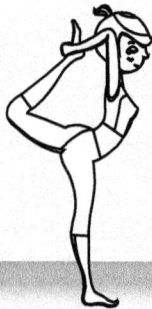

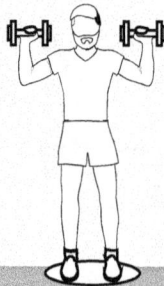

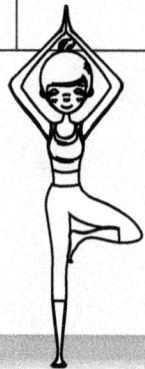

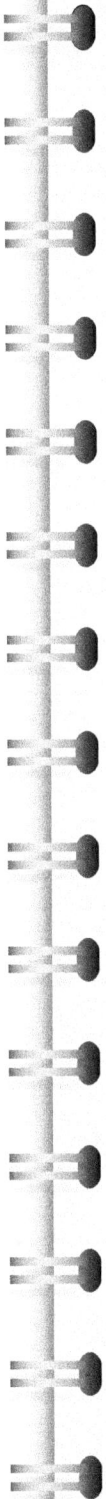

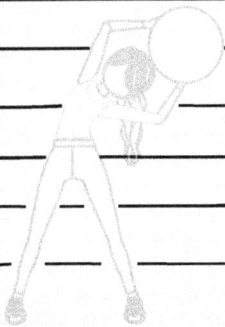

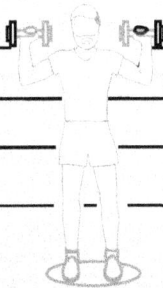

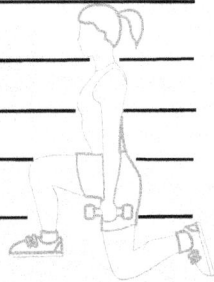

Date:_____

Aerobic / Cardio

Exercises	Time/ Distance	Intensity	Calories Burned

Strenght

Exercises	Sets/ Rep	Weight	Rest

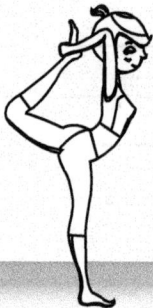

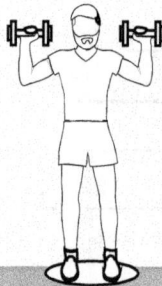

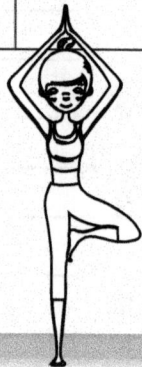

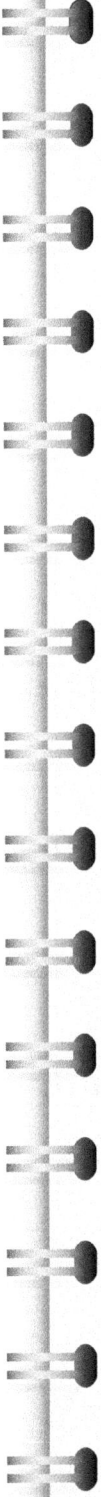

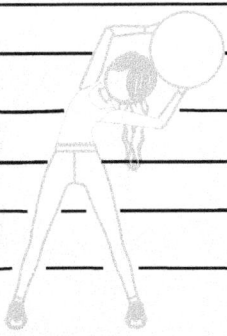

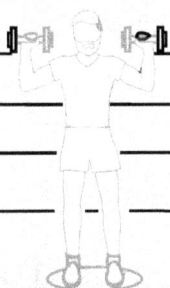

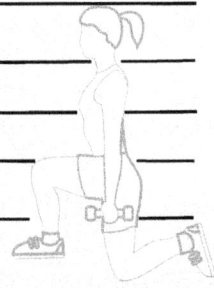

Date:_____

Aerobic /Cardio

Exercises	Time/ Distance	Intensity	Calories Burned

Strenght

Exercises	Sets/ Rep	Weight	Rest

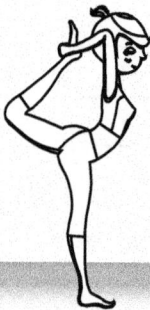

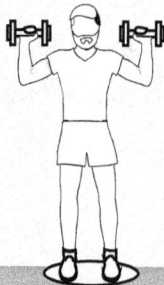

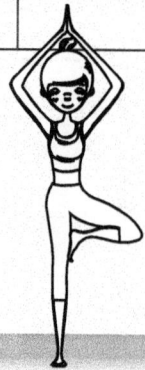

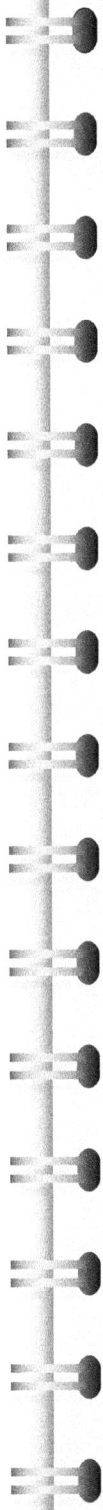
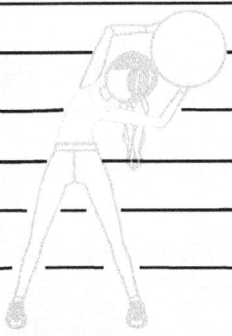
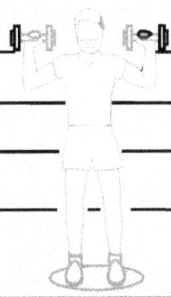
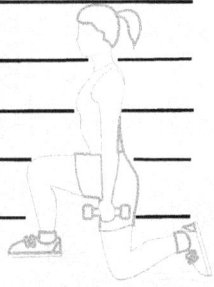

Date:_____

Aerobic /Cardio

Exercises	Time/ Distance	Intensity	Calories Burned

Strenght

Exercises	Sets/ Rep	Weight	Rest

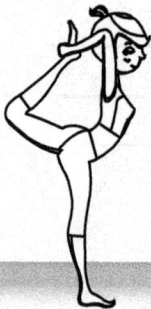

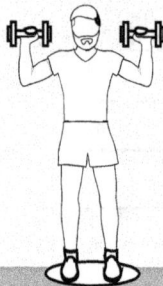

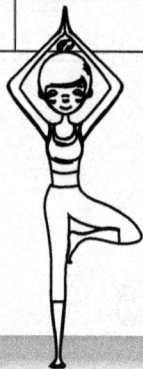

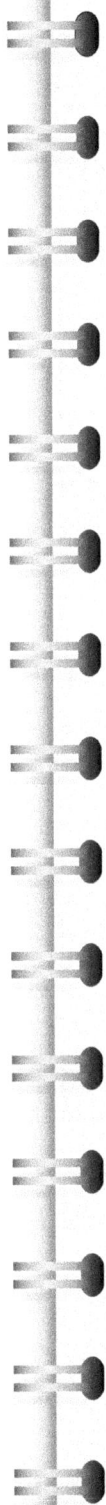

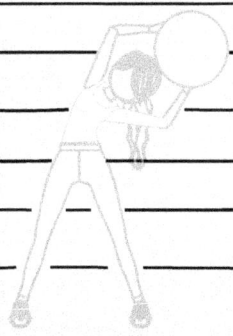

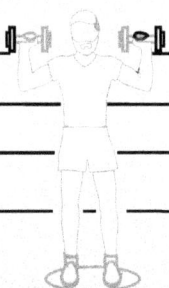

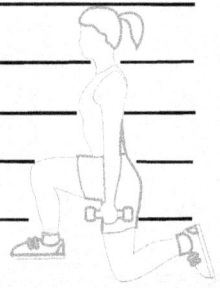

Date:_____

Aerobic /Cardio

Exercises	Time/ Distance	Intensity	Calories Burned

Strenght

Exercises	Sets/ Rep	Weight	Rest

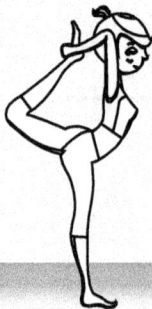

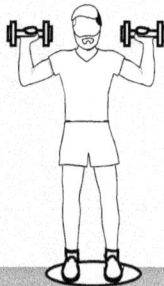

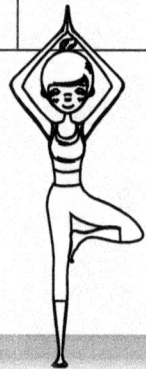

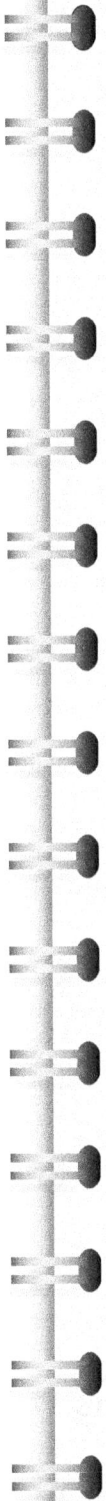

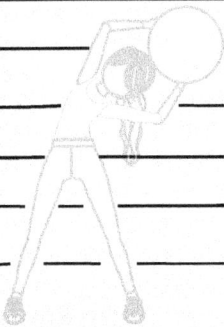

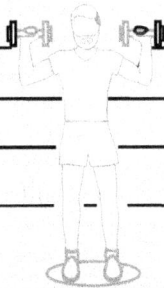

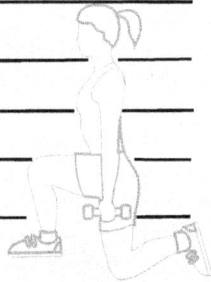

Date:_____

Aerobic /Cardio

Exercises	Time/ Distance	Intensity	Calories Burned

Strenght

Exercises	Sets/ Rep	Weight	Rest

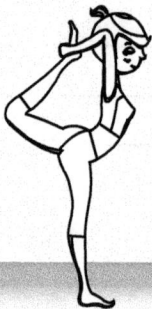

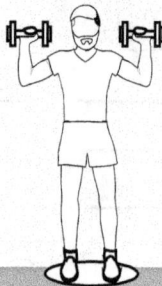

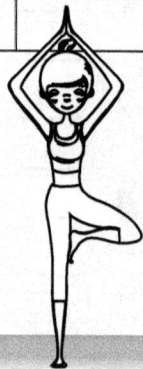

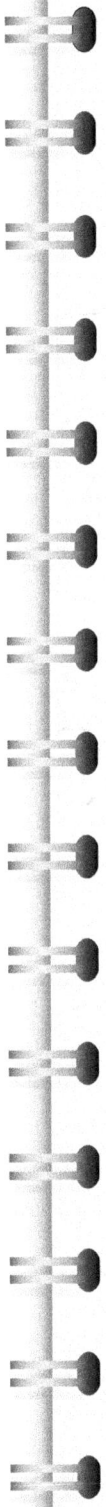

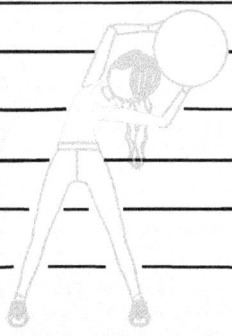

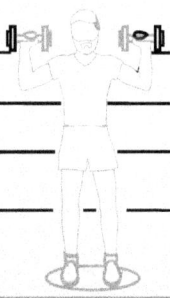

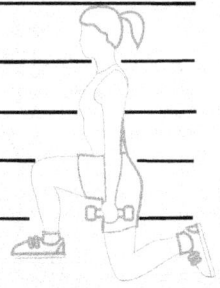

Date:_____

Aerobic /Cardio

Exercises	Time/ Distance	Intensity	Calories Burned

Strenght

Exercises	Sets/ Rep	Weight	Rest

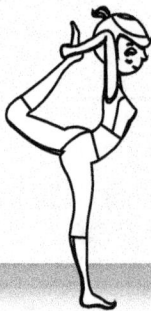

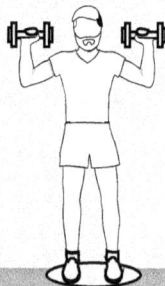

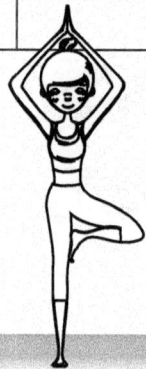

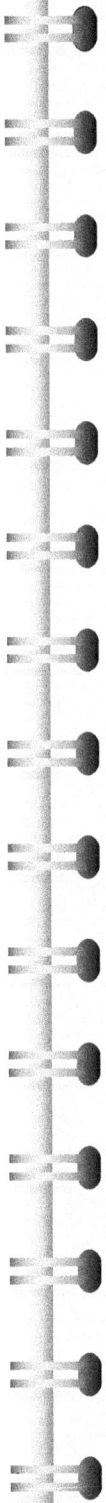
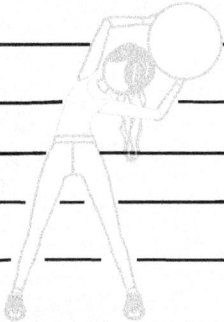
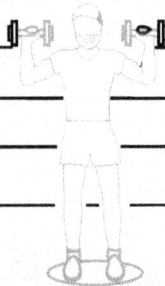
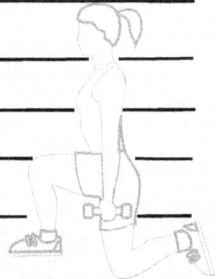

Date:_____

Aerobic /Cardio

Exercises	Time/ Distance	Intensity	Calories Burned

Strenght

Exercises	Sets/ Rep	Weight	Rest

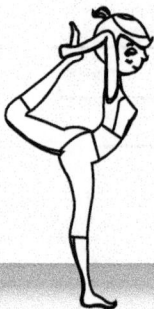

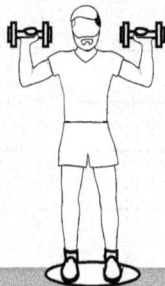

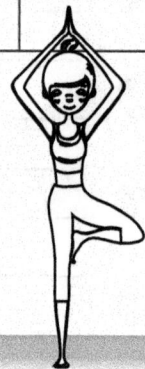

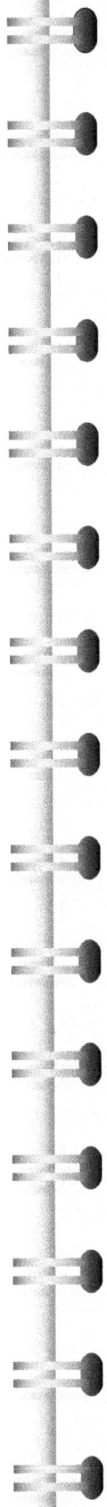

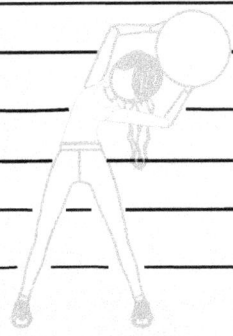

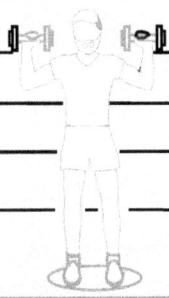

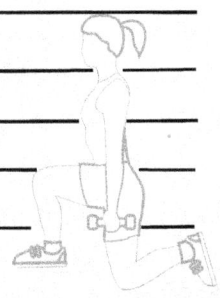

Date:_____

Aerobic /Cardio

Exercises	Time/ Distance	Intensity	Calories Burned

Strenght

Exercises	Sets/ Rep	Weight	Rest

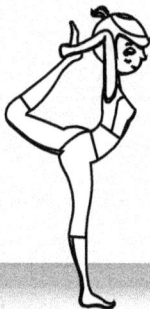

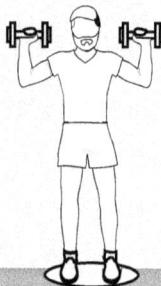

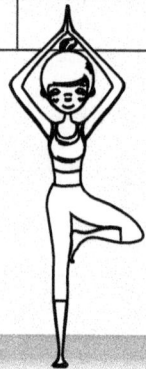

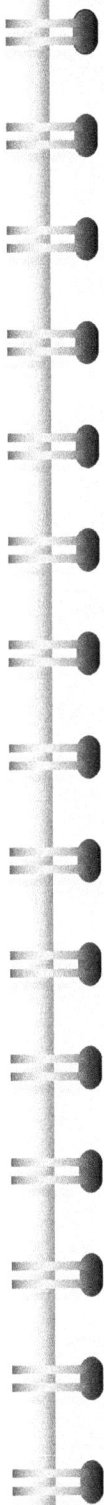

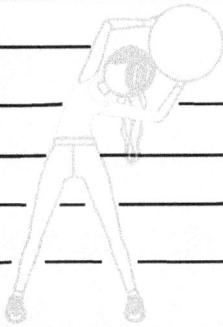

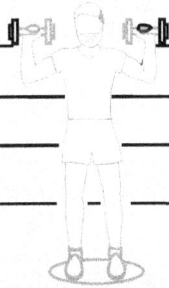

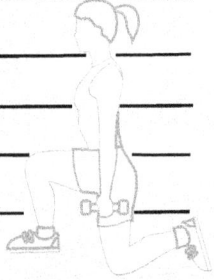

Date:_____

Aerobic /Cardio

Exercises	Time/ Distance	Intensity	Calories Burned

Strenght

Exercises	Sets/ Rep	Weight	Rest

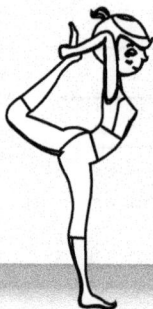

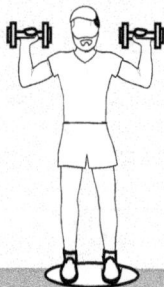

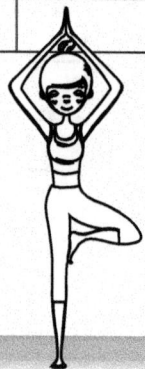

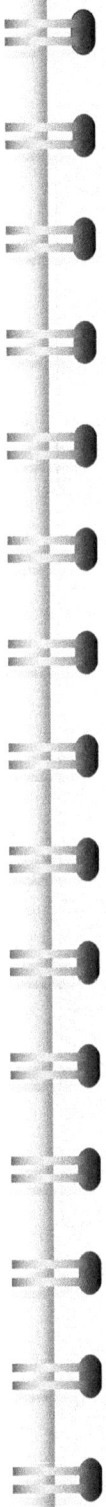

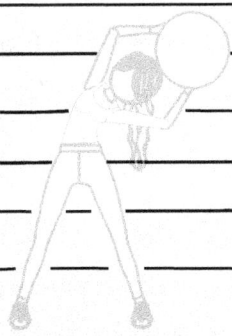

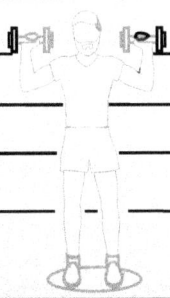

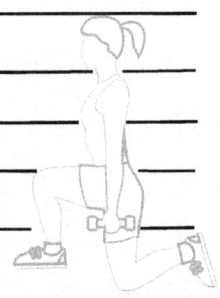

Date:_____

Aerobic /Cardio

Exercises	Time/ Distance	Intensity	Calories Burned

Strenght

Exercises	Sets/ Rep	Weight	Rest

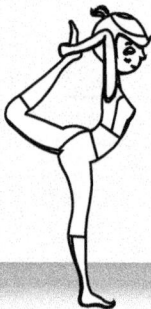

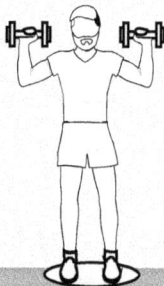

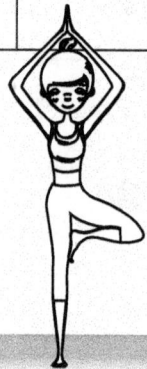

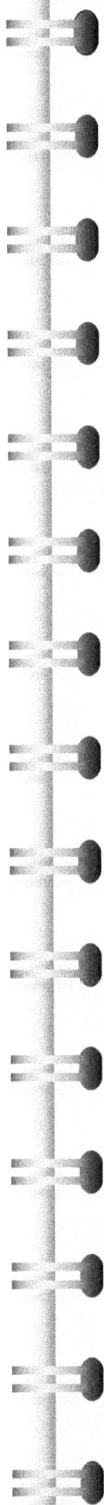

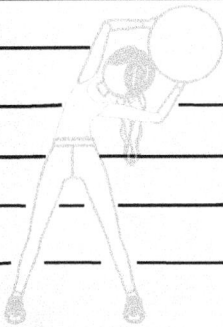

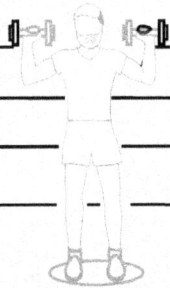

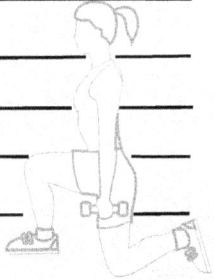

Date:_____

Aerobic / Cardio

Exercises	Time/ Distance	Intensity	Calories Burned

Strenght

Exercises	Sets/ Rep	Weight	Rest

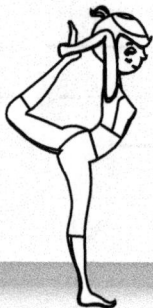

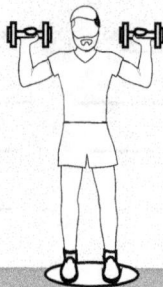

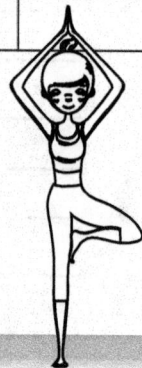

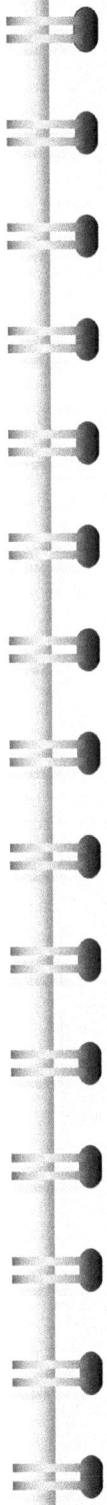

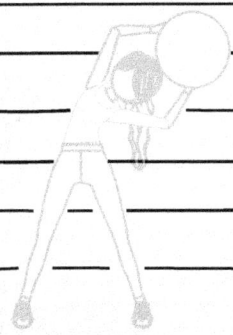

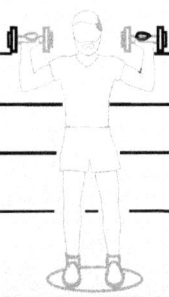

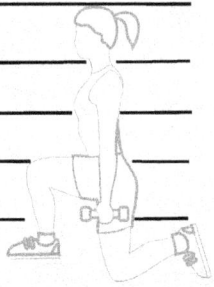

Date:_____

Aerobic /Cardio

Exercises	Time/ Distance	Intensity	Calories Burned

Strenght

Exercises	Sets/ Rep	Weight	Rest

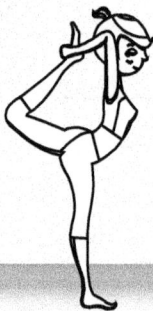

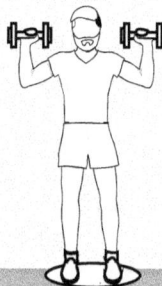

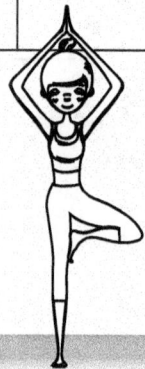

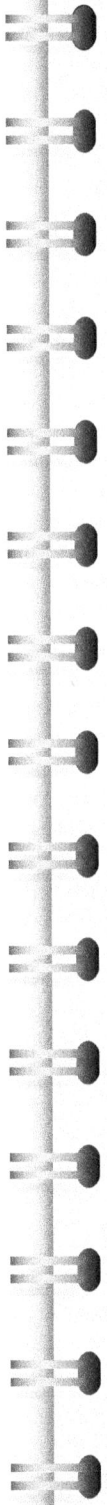

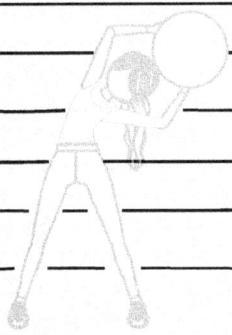
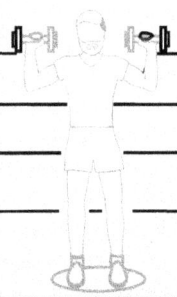
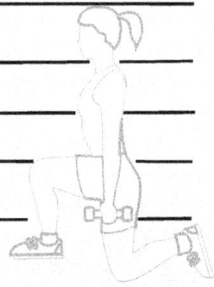

Date:_____

Aerobic /Cardio

Exercises	Time/ Distance	Intensity	Calories Burned

Strenght

Exercises	Sets/ Rep	Weight	Rest

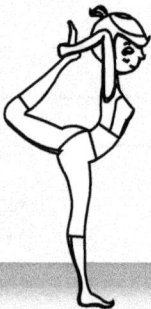

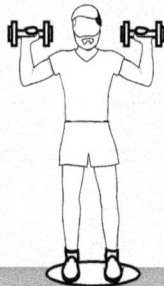

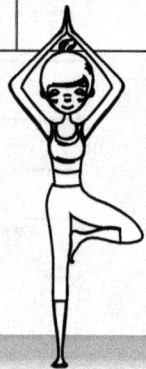

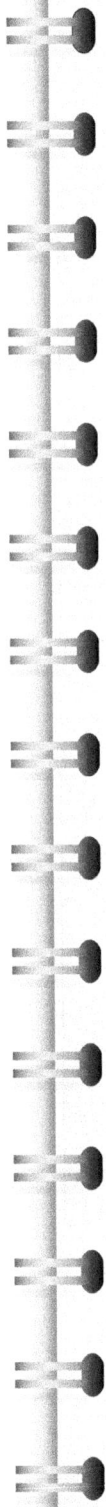

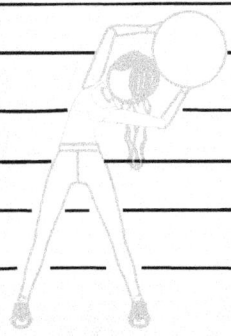

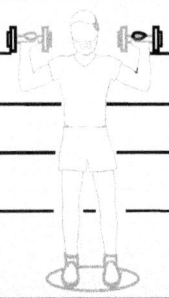

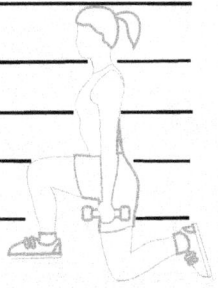

Date:_____

Aerobic /Cardio

Exercises	Time/ Distance	Intensity	Calories Burned

Strenght

Exercises	Sets/ Rep	Weight	Rest

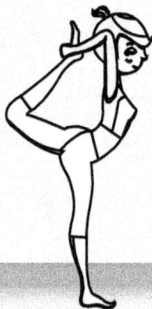

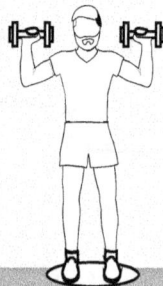

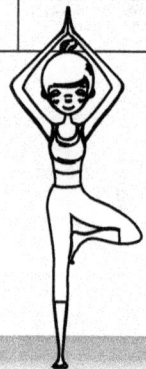

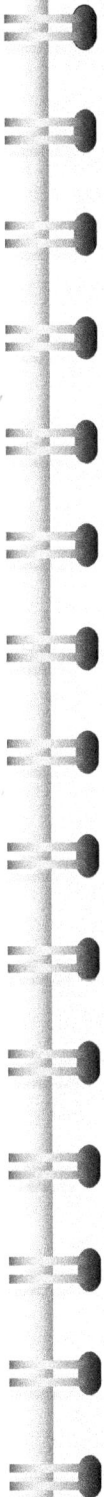

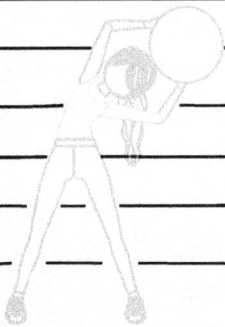

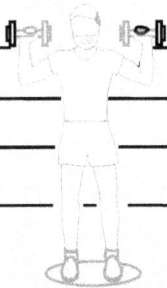

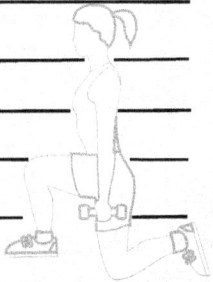

Date:_____

Aerobic /Cardio

Exercises	Time/ Distance	Intensity	Calories Burned

Strenght

Exercises	Sets/ Rep	Weight	Rest

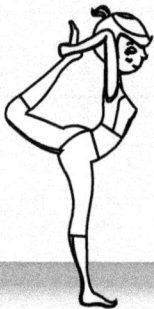

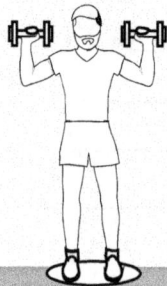

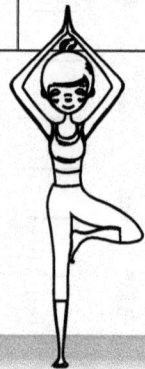

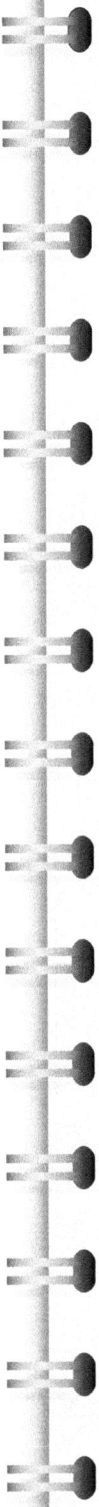

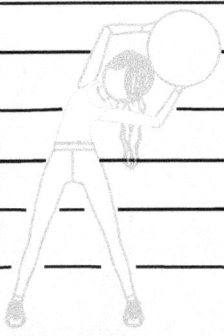

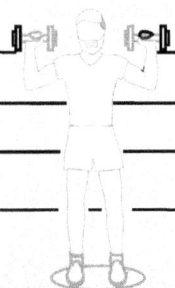

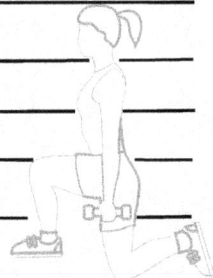

Date:_____

Aerobic /Cardio

Exercises	Time/ Distance	Intensity	Calories Burned

Strenght

Exercises	Sets/ Rep	Weight	Rest

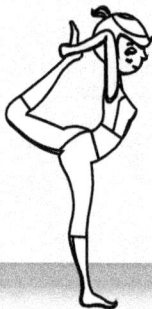

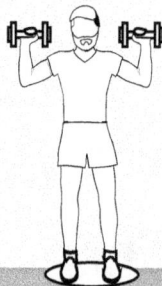

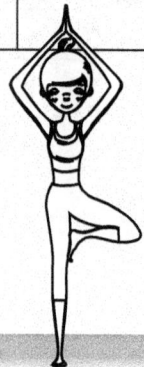

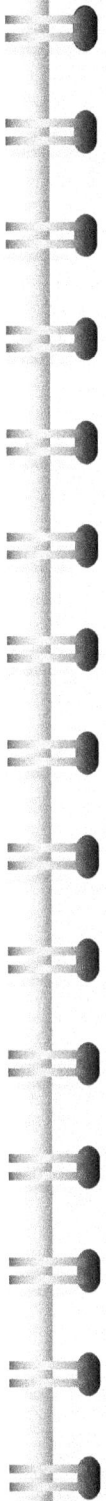

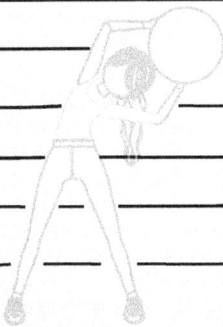

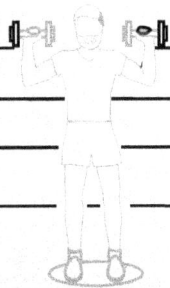

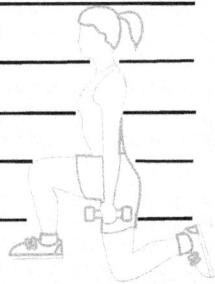

Date:_____

Aerobic /Cardio

Exercises	Time/ Distance	Intensity	Calories Burned

Strenght

Exercises	Sets/ Rep	Weight	Rest

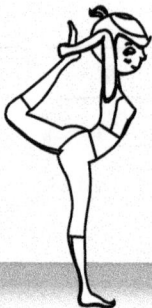

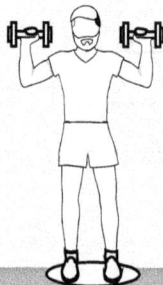

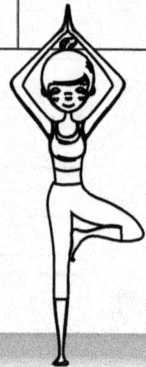

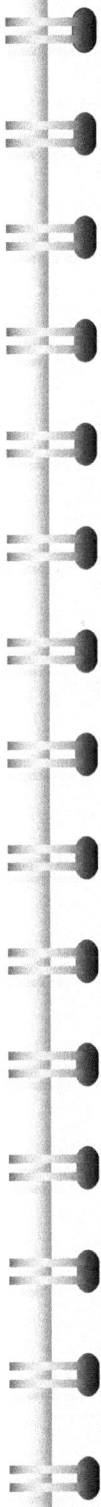

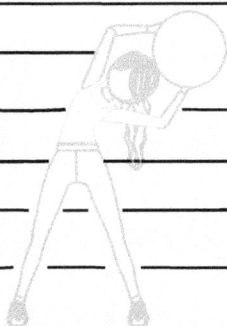

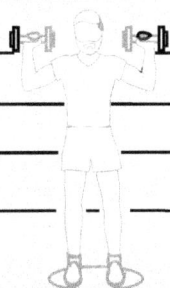

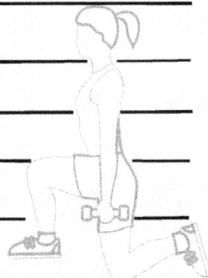

Date:_____

Aerobic /Cardio

Exercises	Time/ Distance	Intensity	Calories Burned

Strenght

Exercises	Sets/ Rep	Weight	Rest

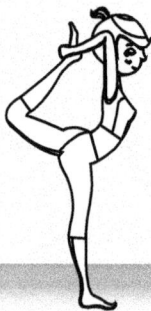

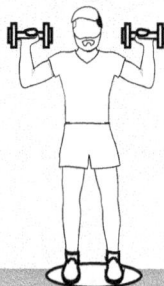

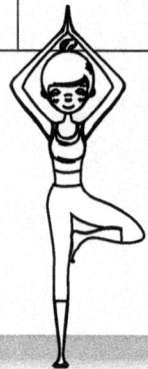

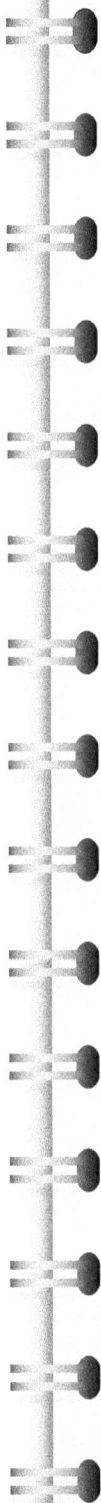

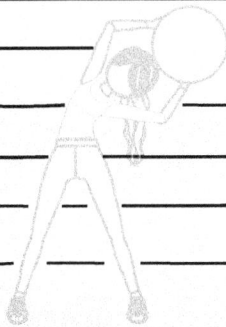

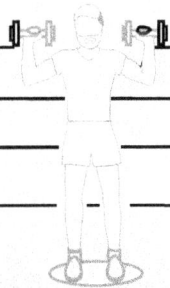

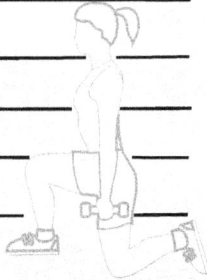

Date:_____

Aerobic / Cardio

Exercises	Time/ Distance	Intensity	Calories Burned

Strenght

Exercises	Sets/ Rep	Weight	Rest

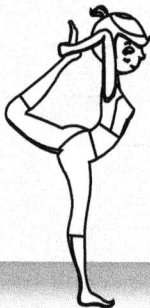

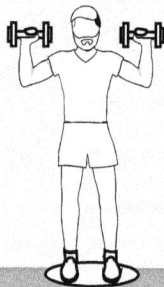

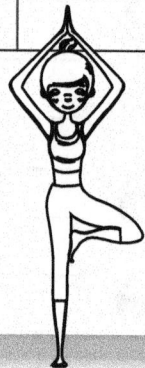

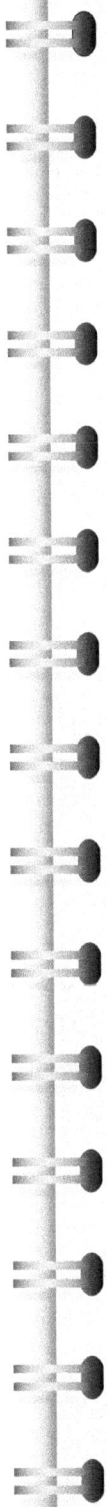

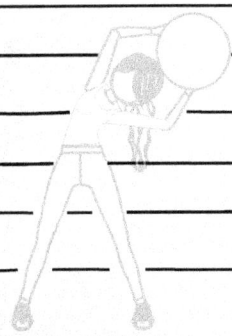

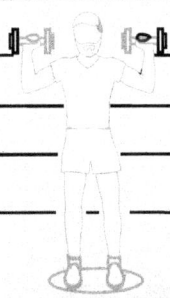

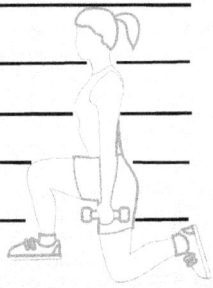

Date:_____

Aerobic /Cardio

Exercises	Time/ Distance	Intensity	Calories Burned

Strenght

Exercises	Sets/ Rep	Weight	Rest

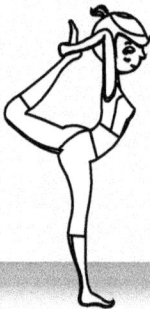

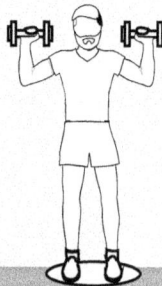

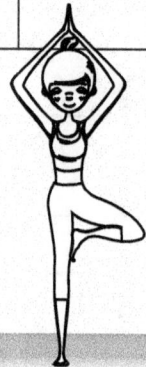

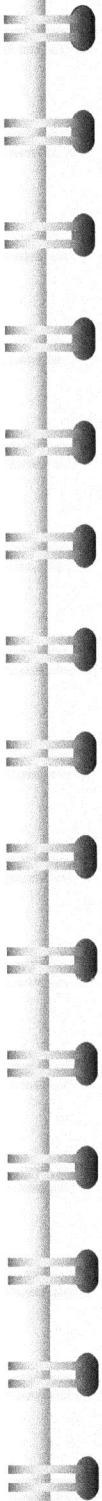

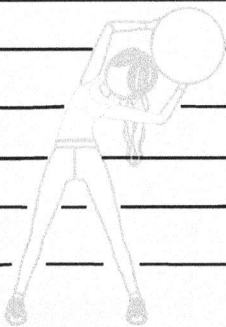

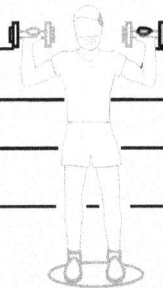

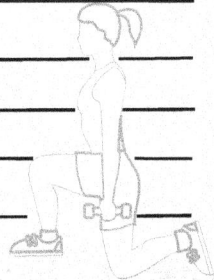

Date:_____

Aerobic / Cardio

Exercises	Time/ Distance	Intensity	Calories Burned

Strenght

Exercises	Sets/ Rep	Weight	Rest

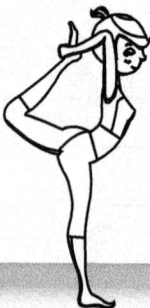

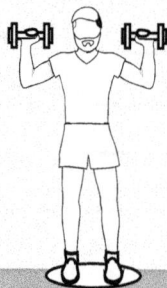

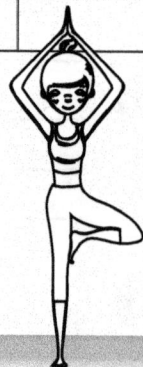

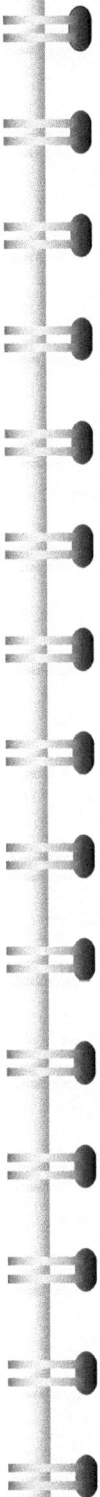

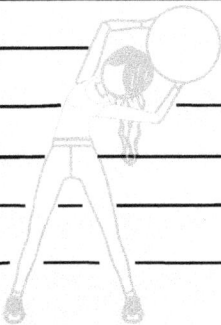

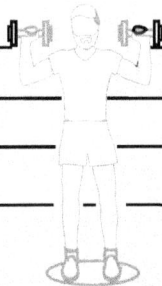

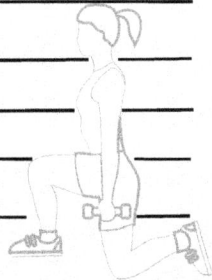

www.ingramcontent.com/pod-product-compliance
Lightning Source LLC
Chambersburg PA
CBHW081419270326
41931CB00015B/3339